Nursing & Health Survival Guide

Research Skills

Jeremy Jolley

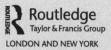

T0033794

Routledge
Taylor & Francis Group

LONDON AND NEW YORK

First published 2013 by Pearson Education Limited

Published 2014 by Routledge
2 Park Square, Milton Park, Abingdon, Oxon OX14 4RN
711 Third Avenue, New York, NY 10017, USA

Routledge is an imprint of the Taylor & Francis Group, an informa business

Copyright © 2013, Taylor & Francis.

The right of Jeremy Jolley to be identified as author of this work has been asserted
by him in accordance with the Copyright, Designs and Patents Act 1988.

All rights reserved. No part of this book may be reprinted or reproduced or utilised in any fo
by him electronic, mechanical, or other means, now known or hereafter invented, including
photocopying and recording, or in any information storage or retrieval system, without perm
in writing from the publishers.

Notices
Knowledge and best practice in this field are constantly changing. As new research and exp
broaden our understanding, changes in research methods, professional practices, or medic
treatment may become necessary.

Practitioners and researchers must always rely on their own experience and knowledge in
evaluating and using any information, methods, compounds, or experiments described here
using such information or methods they should be mindful of their own safety and the safet
others, including parties for whom they have a professional responsibility.

To the fullest extent of the law, neither the Publisher nor the authors, contributors, or editori
assume any liability for any injury and/or damage to persons or property as a matter of proc
liability, negligence or otherwise, or from any use or operation of any methods, products,
instructions, or ideas contained in the material herein.

ISBN 13: 978-0-273-78634-4 (hbk)

British Library Cataloguing-in-Publication Data
A catalogue record for the print edition is available from the British Library

Library of Congress Cataloging-in-Publication Data
Jolley, Jeremy.
    Research skills / Jeremy Jolley.
        p. ; cm. -- (Nursing & health survival guide)
    Includes bibliographical references.
    ISBN 978-0-273-78634-4 (pbk.) -- ISBN 978-0-273-78639-9 (ePub) --
ISBN 978-0-273-78640-5 (eText)
    I. Title. II. Series: Nursing & health survival guides.
    [DNLM: 1. Nursing Research--methods. 2. Data Collection--methods.
3. Research Design. 4. Research. WY 20.5]
    610.73072--dc23

                                                            2012046376

Print edition typeset in 8/9.5pt Helvetica by 35

contents

While effort has been made to ensure that the content
of this guide is accurate, no responsibility will be taken
for inaccuracies, omissions or errors. This is a guide only.
The information is provided solely on the basis that readers
will be responsible for making their own assessment and
adhering to organisation policy of the matters discussed
therein. The author does not accept liability to any person for
the information obtained from this publication or loss or
damages incurred as a result of reliance upon the material
contained in this guide.

Definitions

■ WHAT IS RESEARCH?

Research is any enquiry that is systematic in its nature and which seeks to ensure that the results of that enquiry can be judged by others to be beyond criticism.

Research involves the collection and analysis of 'data'. Data can exist as numbers, words, pictures and anything else that can be collected and subjected to analysis.

The elements of research can be found in everyday life and in clinical practice. We 'research' the market when we buy a new TV or car, or when we try to find out about a disease or treatment that is new to us. Research in the context of this book is fundamentally different from these daily activities only in that:

- The way we go about the research (the design and the method) is identified.
- The way we interpret or analyse the data is documented.
- We document the above expressly so that others can critique our work and so that we can convince them that our research can be trusted (i.e. it is 'robust').

So, research:

- Is systematic. Data is collected and analysed using a stated method; that method is not ad hoc, it does not use trial and error.
- Involves the collection of data. The data can be new data, data which already exists or data that someone else has used in their research but the data is always 'raw'. Raw data is original data, not summaries of data.

A library search and a literature review are *not* research because they do not seek to find raw data.

■ THE PURPOSE OF RESEARCH

- To generate new knowledge
- To enable a new interpretation of existing data

■ EVIDENCE-BASED PRACTICE (EBP)

This is a broader term than 'research'. EBP is an acknowledgement that:

- Clinical practice must sometimes take place even where research is not available.
- There are 'other' (non-research) forms of evidence which do have value.

Acceptable forms of non-research evidence

Peer review	Allows for a formal process whereby fellow professionals can review ideas for practice development
Clinical audit	A process by which practice can be met against defined standards
Benchmarking	Where practice can be mapped against agreed definitions of best practice – often between different institutions
Established clinical expertise	Is valuable, especially where success and failure rates are known
Tradition	What practitioners have always done may be flawed but is still likely to be effective

Policy and guidelines	Have been subject to careful planning and peer review
Anecdotal evidence	Evidence that does not meet the criteria for 'research' but can still be documented and subjected to review

Non-acceptable forms of evidence

Intuition	Intuition is an unreasoned belief in something (a feeling that x = y). Evidence for this belief cannot be provided by the individual and cannot be shared with others
Trial and error	Is haphazard, non-systematic and difficult to record and report to others
Unpublished work (including unpublished research)	Has not been made subject to peer review

■ THE KNOWLEDGE HIERARCHY

1. Research
2. Benchmarking or audit against evidence-based criteria
3. Policy and guidelines supported by evidence
4. Tradition and clinical expertise

It is important to remember that research provides the best quality of evidence and that we should only use other forms of evidence when research is not available.

■ QUANTITATIVE AND QUALITATIVE RESEARCH

| Quantitative | Deals with quantities (counts) of things and usually involves numbers. Usually adopts the positivist paradigm (traditional science) and relates to objective and measurable phenomena |
| Qualitative | Deals with the quality of things and usually involves words (sometimes drawings, music, etc.). Usually adopts the constructivist paradigm which focuses on human experience and the interpretation of it |

■ THE RESEARCH PROCESS

Whatever form research takes, it is always systematic and follows this process:

The hunch	A gut feeling about a possible enquiry or the realisation that knowledge is needed where it is currently absent
Review of the existing literature	To find out what is already known and what still needs to be found out
Problem identification	This 'problem' is the thing that the research will aim to solve. Sometimes this is formulated as a hypothesis, sometimes as a 'research question'
Plan for research (design and method)	The research is planned to produce a design and method aimed to enable the research to be successful
Data collection	The data is collected

Data analysis	The data is analysed, often using statistics (quantitative research) or interpretive analysis (qualitative research)
Discussion of results/evaluation	The results (findings) of the research are exposed to critique. The implications of the findings are discussed
Publication	The research is published in order to make it available to peer review

The literature

It is important to use only the professional or academic literature.

Professional and academic literature:

- Is written using an accepted standard of language that is respectful of both the subject matter and other academics/professionals
- Employs language that is non-emotional and objective
- Is focused on the subject in question
- Contains both analysis and synthesis, that is, it 'questions' and it deals with conflicting arguments, ideas or evidence
- Is made subject to peer review.

There are two main types of literature:

- research – describes a research study
- anecdotal – not research but useful for background 'ideas'.

■ ONLINE DATABASES

Cinahl*	http://www.ebscohost.com/academic/cinahl-plus-with-full-text/
Cochrane library*	http://www.thecochranelibrary.com
Academic Search Complete*	http://www.ebscohost.com/academic/academic-search-complete
Medline*	http://www.ebscohost.com/academic/medline-with-full-text
National Institute for Health and Clinical Excellence (NICE)	http://www.nice.org.uk/
Evidence in Health and Social Care†	https://www.evidence.nhs.uk/

* Most universities offer these databases – access these via your university library website.
† A useful source of free information for any NHS employee, allows free access to Cinahl, Medline, Cochrane.

■ USING DATABASES EFFECTIVELY

- Keep notes of your search strategy.
- Always tick the 'peer reviewed' box.
- Select the 'publication type' to 'research'; options to search for particular types of research such as double-blind control trials, may also be available.
- Consider selecting the 'full text' option to save time in finding and ordering articles via your library.
- Consider confining the date of publication to (for example) the past 10 years.

■ TYPES OF DISCUSSION

- **Description:** to clarify what research has already been undertaken and to summarise the literature.
- **Analysis:** to interpret, question or judge the 'worth' of the material and how relevant it is to the focus of your own work.
- **Synthesis:** to deal with unanswered questions. In research, it is often the case that two or more research projects seem to have conflicting 'findings'; it is necessary to 'deal' with this and to make judgements on what may cause this conflict.

■ HOW TO REVIEW THE LITERATURE

- Identify a clear objective.
- Work within your resources (time).
- Identify what kind of literature you are looking for:
  - research
  - anecdotal
  - existing review of the literature
  - books.
- Identify the academic level of journal you are aiming at.
- Get help from a librarian, library guides, etc.
- Make notes on everything you read.
- For the research literature, try to identify:
  - What was the aim of the research?
  - What was planned to be done (the research method)?
  - How was it done (the intervention or techniques such as interviews or questionnaires)?
  - What was found?
- For anecdotal literature, try to identify:
  - What was the focus of the paper?
  - What was described?

- What were the authors arguing?
- How was the argument supported?
- Is their argument credible?
- Be prepared to read and re-read your literature.

■ WRITING YOUR ACCOUNT

- You should make your own arguments and use the literature to support your arguments.
- Create a plan:
  - Your introduction to the topic
  - What arguments will you try to make
  - How can you use the literature you have found to support your arguments
  - What your conclusions will be.
- Try to use description (in your introduction), analysis and synthesis.
- Try to make your discussion flow logically.

■ EDITING YOUR WORK

Editing your essay can take longer than writing the first draft, so ask yourself the following questions:

- Is my account clear, is it understandable?
- Is my English clear?
- What am I arguing?
- Are my arguments logical ordered?
- Have I provided an analysis?
- Where the literature is complex or where it suggests different things, have I synthesised these elements?
- Is my account interesting?
- Does my account add something to the literature I have read?

Your account should?
- Communicate an argument (have a common trajectory, flows well)
- Be questioning (analysis)
- Come to a conclusion (synthesis).

Further reading

Cronin, P. *et al.* (2008). 'Undertaking a literature review: a step-by-step approach', *British Journal of Nursing (BJN)*, 17(1): 38–43.

Common quantitative designs

Quantitative research exists in two main forms:

Descriptive (retrospective)	Looks at what is or what was
Experimental (prospective)	Looks at what might be (an experiment)

Research can be classified according to the amount of control exerted over the variables being studied:

Randomisation	Applied to sampling and/or allocation to groups
Control	The provision of a group which was not exposed to the intervention
Blinding	Keeping information on group allocation or type of intervention hidden from those who will provide and collect the data

■ SAMPLING

Probability (random) sampling

Simple random sampling	Using a random number generator
Systematic sampling	For example, every tenth name or making an observation every 15 minutes
Stratified random sample	Ensures equal representation of sub-classes, e.g. males and females
Cluster sampling	Geographical selection (three hospitals)
Mixed sampling	Simply a mixture of two or more of the above

Non-probability (non-random) sampling

Purposive sampling (judgement sampling)	Subjects are selected because the researcher believes that they are representative
Convenience sampling	Selecting people who happen to be available
Quota sampling	Convenience sampling with controls to ensure equal representation of sub-groups
Volunteers	Subjects choose to be included

■ RECRUITMENT (SAMPLING) IN QUALITATIVE RESEARCH

Participants must meet the following criteria (Magilvy and Thomas, 2009):

- *Have experienced* the phenomenon under examination
- Are *able* to communicate their experiences to the researcher
- Are *willing* to communicate their experiences.

■ INDEPENDENT AND DEPENDENT VARIABLES

The independent variable is designed to cause an effect which is measured in the dependent variable.

Examples of groups (conditions) and independent and dependent variables

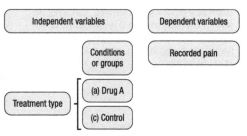

In the above, the effect of the independent variable, 'treatment type' is measured in the dependent variables, 'recorded pain'.

■ DESIGNS

In the illustrations given below 'X' is the intervention and '0' represents a research group.

Survey
A survey has just one descriptive group.

One group post-test only design
$\times 0$
The intervention is given and the effect determined
Problem – it is not known if the effect was already present prior to the intervention.

One group pre-test post-test
0×0
This adds a pre-test (good). However, we cannot tell whether the effect was due to the pre-testing or the intervention (or both). Sometimes pre-testing can lead to participants feeling that they are cared about, causing an unwanted effect.

Two group post-test only
$\times 0_1$
$\quad 0_2$
This is a common design. However, it lacks pre-testing.

Two group, before/after design
$0_1 \times 0_2$
$0_1 \quad 0_2$
This is frequently used in medicine in randomised control trials. It is a good design. However, it does not tell us if

pre-testing caused an effect, nor whether time itself had an effect.

The Solomon four group design

$) \times 0$
$)\quad 0$
$\quad \times 0$
$\qquad 0$

This is an 'exhaustive' design which both allows for the effect of pre-testing to be measured and also the effect of 'time'. (Would the effect have happened anyway?)

Further reading

Edmonds, W. A. and Kennedy, T. D. (2012). *An applied reference guide to research designs: quantitative, qualitative, and mixed methods*, Los Angeles: Sage Publications.

McGahee, T. W. and Tingen, M. S. (2009). 'The use of the Solomon four-group design in nursing research', *Southern Online Journal of Nursing Research*, 9(1): 4.

Data collection methods

COMMON DATA COLLECTION METHODS

- Questionnaire
- Interview
- Participant and non-participant observation
- Focus groups
- Existing data
- Historical data
- Audio, film and photographic records

Questionnaire

Can deal with the following kinds of data:

- Facts as categories (yes, no, blue, has pain)
- Impressions as a scale (e.g. pain scale)
- Open-ended questions.

Can be delivered:

- Via a website
- By post
- At a one-to-one meeting with the participant.

The questionnaire can be inexpensive and efficient. However, it is hard to ensure that participants properly understand the questions, and that they try to answer truthfully and fully. Open-ended questions do not allow probing and are difficult to analyse.

Interview

Can be used to collect factual data (e.g. age, sex) but is also useful for longer dialogues. Interviews are the main form of data collection in qualitative studies.

Difficulties include the fact that it is more difficult to recruit participants to interviews and interviews are resource intensive. Conducting an interview well takes experience and requires good communication skills. Probing skills (for deeper or emotionally sensitive dialogue) also take time to learn.

Different types of probes (Whiting 2008, p. 38):

- Silence – allows the participant to think
- Echo – the researcher repeats what the participant has said in order to encourage elaboration
- Verbal agreement – as in, 'yes, I understand, go on . . .'

- 'Tell me more' – the interviewer directly asks the participant to expand the detail
- Leading – asks a question which leads in a particular direction
- Baiting – gives the impression of being aware of something the participant is referring to and tends to encourage further discourse on the matter.

Participant and non-participant observation
This is sometimes used in qualitative studies but is only rarely used in quantitative studies. The researcher is able to see 'real' practice. However, people can change their practice while being watched (Hawthorn effect) and objectively measuring what is seen can be challenging.

Focus groups
Often used in qualitative studies, a focus group is essentially an interview with a group of people. It is used where interaction between group members enhances the depth of data elicited. It is not a shortcut to doing several one-to-one interviews.

Existing data
Data already exists in, for example, hospital records, diaries and the census.

Historical data
Usually used in research into the history of healthcare. Historians often use existing archives (hospital archives) to obtain historical documents such as letters and reports. Historians also use 'oral histories', essentially interviews with older people about their memories of events in the past.

Audio, film and photographic records

It is important to understand that 'data' can exist in many different forms. These forms of data are not much used in healthcare research but may be used in historical research studies.

Further reading

Banner, D. J. (2010). 'Qualitative interviewing: preparation for practice', *Canadian Journal of Cardiovascular Nursing*, 20(3): 27–30.

McKnight, M. (2006). 'The information seeking of on-duty critical care nurses: evidence from participant observation and in-context interviews', *Journal of the Medical Library Association*, 94(2): 145–151.

Meadows, K. A. (2003). 'So you want to do research? 5: questionnaire design', *British Journal of Community Nursing*, 8(12): 562–570.

Nicholl, H. (2010). 'Diaries as a method of data collection in research', *Paediatric Nursing*, 22(7): 16–20.

Rothwell, E. (2010). 'Analyzing focus group data: content and interaction', *Journal for Specialists in Pediatric Nursing*, 15(2): 176–180.

Sweeney, J. F. (2005). 'Historical research: examining documentary sources', *Nurse Researcher*, 12(3): 61–73.

Types of data

■ NUMERICAL (QUANTITATIVE) DATA

Levels of measurement

LEVEL	FORM	EXAMPLES
Nominal	Categories	Yes/No Blue/Red/Yellow Male/Female
Ordinal	Short scale or ranked data	1–5 Likert scale 1–10 Pain scale
Interval	Long (continuous) scale	Exam marks 1–100
Ratio	Long (continuous) scale with no parameters	Pulse rate Blood pressure

Levels of measurement are important because:
- They help to determine the appropriate statistical test.
- Interval and ratio data are 'richer'; they contain more information.

A question yielding nominal data (categories)

Are you:

Male	
Female	

A question yielding ordinal data

Statement: I like Likert scales

Strongly agree	Agree	Undecided	Disagree	Strongly Disagree
5	4	3	2	1

The original 'ordinal' scale consisted of a list of things in 'order'. We cannot place in order lots of things, so an ordinal scale is always short.

The ordinal scale is not continuous (interval level) because '2.5' may be meaningful but cannot be selected.

A question yielding interval data

Your exam mark (1–100)

The 'ends' of the scale are limited at 1 and 100.

A question yielding ratio data

Systolic blood pressure

The scale has no limits.

■ TYPES OF QUALITATIVE DATA

- Spoken word
- Documents
- Participant observation
- Non-participant observation
- Video/film

- Photographs
- Drawings

Probability and significance

It is usually the case that statistical analysis is run in order to calculate the probability of an effect being due to chance alone. This is often referred to as 'significance'.

Probability is usually abbreviated to 'p. x'. So that:

p. = 0.10 means 10% or 10:100 (non-significant)

p. = 0.05 means 5% or 5:100

p. = 0.01 means 1% or 1:100

p. = 0.001 means 0.1% or 1:1000

Definition of probability

- Chance is that part of the objective and measurable world that is unknown.
- In research, an intervention may produce an effect. However, 'chance' can also produce an effect.
- Statistical procedures try to measure the risk that chance might have caused the effect. This is expressed as probability (p.).
- We may be satisfied that if the probability is less than 5% (p. = 0.05), the effect was probably caused by the intervention and not by chance.

Probability and significance need to be open to judgement, so that:

- p. = 0.05 may be regarded as significant where the results of the study, if implemented, would not create a life or death situation.

- Research on a new drug is likely to want to see a greater level of significance than $p. = 0.05$.

Variance

All variables (things we can measure) 'vary' (have variance). A person's systolic BP may not be the same, even when it is taken on three occasions, 2 minutes apart. The three results will be similar but not identical: BP is a 'variable', that is, it varies. Variance is normal.

Determining probability

Statistical tests usually determine probability by:

1. Determining the variability within each group of data (each 'condition')
2. Determining the variability between the groups (conditions)
3. Where the variability within each group is greater than the variability between the groups then the result will tend to be non-significant
4. Where the variability within each group is less than the variability between the groups then the result will tend to be 'significant'.

Caution

Statistics is not about 'proof'. Even if the result is $p. < 0.00000001$, there is still a 'risk' (a small one) that the effect was caused by chance.

Selecting the right statistical procedure

■ DESCRIPTIVE STATISTICS

These are used to describe and summarise data.

Mean	Average value
Median	The middle value in a range
Mode	The most commonly occurring value
Variance	A measure of the degree to which the data varies (degree of dispersion around the mean)
Standard deviation	A measure of variance which can be used to compare the variance of two or more variables

■ INFERENTIAL STATISTICS

These are used to draw 'inferences' from the data and are associated with identifying probability.

In order to select the most appropriate statistical procedure it is necessary to consider the following factors about the data and the design of the study:

1. Types of variables

Is the data:

- Nominal
- Ordinal
- Interval or ratio?

2. Number of variables

- How many independent variables are there?
- How many dependant variables are there?

3. Related or unrelated design
- Related – data is collected from the same participant on two or more occasions
- Unrelated – data is collected from different participants

4. Differences and correlations
Does the study deal with:
- Differences or
- Correlations?

5. Parametric and non-parametric
Does the data meet the criteria (assumptions) for a parametric statistical procedure? These assumptions are that:
- Data is normally distributed
- The variances should be similar
- The data must be interval or ratio.

Non-parametric tests can be run on almost any data (no data 'assumptions' are needed). Parametric tests, however, can only be run on data which meets the assumptions given above.

Statistics for nominal data

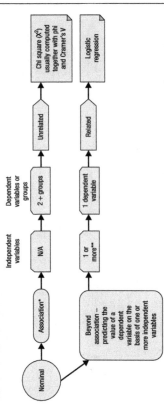

Nominal → Association* → N/A → 2 + groups → Unrelated → Chi square (χ^2) usually computed together with phi and Cramer's V

Nominal → Beyond association — predicting the value of a dependent variable on the basis of one or more independent variables → 1 or more** → 1 dependent variable → Related → Logistic regression

Independent variables

Dependent variables or groups

* 'Association' is a kind of middle-term between 'differences' and 'correlation' but which doesn't quite mean 'correlation'. It is commonly used for 'differences' but is also used where the lack of 'difference' can be meaningful (association). Phi and Cramer's V are specifically used to measure whether one variable is 'associated' with another variable. Chi square itself is chiefly used where 'differences' are expected. In practice, chi square, phi and Cramer's V tend to be calculated at the same time.

** The independent variable (sometimes here called a 'predictor variable') can be nominal data or may exist as a scale. The dependent variable in logistic regression will be nominal (categories).

Non-parametric statistics for ordinal data

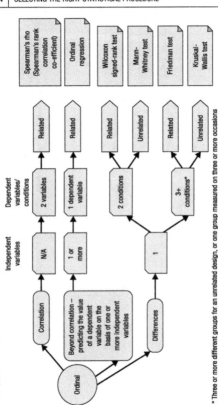
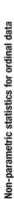

* Three or more different groups for an unrelated design, or one group measured on three or more occasions

Parametric statistics for interval and ratio data: correlations and predictions

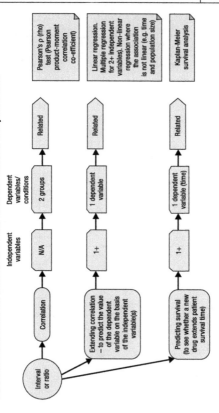

Parametric statistics for interval and ratio data: differences

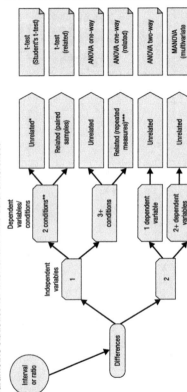

* Unrelated, sometimes referred to as 'unpaired' or 'independent samples'.

** Two groups or, for a related design, one group measured on two occasions.

*** For a related design, the independent variable is often 'time'. The dependent variable consists of measures taken from one group (one

Further reading

Scott, I. and Mazhindu, D. (2005). *Statistics for health care professionals*, Los Angeles: Sage Publications.

Commonly used statistical tests

Analysis of variance (ANOVA)	A range of parametric statistical procedures designed to be run on interval and ratio data. Generally used to identify the effect of one or more independent variables on one or more dependent variables in a manner that we would be likely to see in an experiment or clinical trial
Chi square (X^2) (Pearson chi square)	Pearson chi square is used for nominal data (categories) where associations are hypothesised.
Confidence interval	A confidence interval is a measure of how likely it is that a measure (e.g. the mean) taken from a sample would be found in the population
Cronbach's alpha	Used to test internal consistency or reliability. It is most commonly used to test that a questionnaire is 'reliable'
Friedman	A non-parametric equivalent of the one-way analysis of variance for a related design. The Freidman test is run where there is one variable which is measured on more than two occasions

Normality tests (Kolmogorov-Smirnov test and Shapiro-Wilk)	Used to test that data is normally distributed – a condition of using parametric tests such as ANOVA
Kruskal-Wallis	A non-parametric equivalent of the one-way analysis of variance for unrelated groups. There should be one independent variable with more than two conditions
Mann-Whitney	A non-parametric equivalent of the t-test for unrelated groups. There needs to be one independent variable with two conditions
MANOVA (Multivariate analysis of variance)	MANOVA is an extension of ANOVA. It can deal with more than one independent variable and more than one dependent variable. MANOVA is used in situations that are essentially 'multivariate'
Mean (arithmetic mean)	A summary measure of interval and ratio data; the average value
Median	The median is the middle score of ordinal data. The median of 12, 23, 34, 45, 56, 67, 78, 89, 100 is 56
Mode	The most frequently occurring score. Mode is most commonly used for categorical (nominal data)
Odds ratio	Odds ratio is used in Cochrane systematic reviews. It is used in the meta-analysis of data combined from several studies

One-way ANOVA (unrelated)	A parametric test used where differences are hypothesised and where there is one independent variable containing more than two conditions. The groups of data must be unrelated
One-way ANOVA (related)	A parametric test, used where differences are hypothesised, where there is one independent variable and where participants are exposed to the testing on more than two occasions. The design must be 'related' (e.g. the same participants are tested on more than two occasions)
Pearson rho (ρ)	The Pearson rho is a parametric correlation test. It is used to identify correlations between two variables where data is at the interval or ratio level of measurement
Regression analysis	Regression procedures (such as 'linear regression') aim to determine if one variable (the predictor variable) has an effect on the other variable (the dependent variable). Regression analysis was originally developed as an extension of correlational analysis. Forms of regression analysis are available for nominal, ordinal and interval data

Shapiro-Wilk	Used to test that data is normally distributed, this being one of the criteria for using parametric statistical tests
Spearman correlation	This is a non-parametric equivalent of Pearson's correlation. It is used where is hypothesised that two variables are correlated
Standard deviation	Standard deviation is a measure of dispersion around the mean or the within-group variability
Survival analysis	These are a range of statistical procedures, including the Kaplan-Meier survival procedure designed to identify the impact of an independent variable on 'survival'. The survival variable is time
t-test	The t-test is a parametric test used to compare the effect of two conditions (one independent variable) and where the design is 'unrelated'
t-test (related) or paired samples t-test	The t-test (related) is a parametric test used to compare the effect of the independent variable on the dependent variable as measured on two occasions. There must be two sets of data taken from the same participants (or matched participants) on two occasions

Two-way ANOVA	A two-way ANOVA is similar to a one-way ANOVA except that it can handle two independent variables. It is a parametric test and is used where there are two independent variables, each with one or more conditions (groups) and one dependent variable
Wilcoxon	The Wilcoxon signed-ranks test is a non-parametric equivalent of the related t-test. It is used where there is one independent variable with two conditions (groups) and where the design is related. In practice, there will be two sets of data taken on two occasions from either the same participants (on both of the two occasions) or from 'matched' participants.

Statistical analysis using SPSS

SPSS is the most widely used statistical software. Most universities and many NHS Trusts provide access to SPSS. Information about SPSS can be found at http://www-01.ibm.com/software/analytics/spss/

SPSS looks rather like a spreadsheet. The columns contain the variables and the rows contain the cases.

SPSS

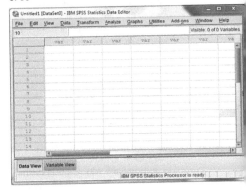

To use SPSS:
1. First, set up the variables, click on 'variable view':

SPSS (variable view)

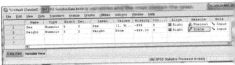

2. In the variable view, add the details of each variable.

. Now go to 'data view' and begin entering the raw data for each variable:

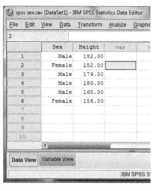

. Now save the file and run the analysis. Go to 'Analyze' and (in this example) select the t-test (independent samples):

Independent sample T-test

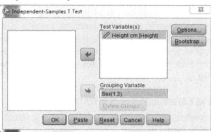

5. Select the test variable (height) and the grouping variable (sex) and press OK and view the results.

Resuit view of SPSS

Sex	N	Mean	Std. Deviation
Male	4	176.5000	7.76745
Female	2	154.0000	2.82843

df	Sig. (2-tailed)
4	.019
3.965	.007

Further reading

Pallant, J. (2010). *SPSS survival manual: a step by step guide to data analysis using SPSS*. Milton Keynes: Open University Press.

Qualitative research

Qualitative research deals with data that cannot easily be quantified but where there is an attempt to capture the richness of human experience. Qualitative research is usua explorative and inductive: that is, it asks questions where th range of available answers is not known. For example, we cannot ask, 'Is it (a), (b) or (c)?' because we do not know what (a), (b), etc. are.

■ KEY APPROACHES IN QUALITATIVE RESEARCH

In practice, the difference between the following approache is quite minor:

Ethnography	Derived from anthropology, focuses on cultural meanings. How the organisation of society is achieved and the meaning people find in their culture or society
Phenomenology	Focuses on the interpretation of the 'lived experience' of individuals
Grounded theory	Focuses on generating theory on social processes by inductive examination of human experience. It is characterised by a close examination of the data together with reflection on the way it is being coded (constant comparative analysis). In practice, it is a relatively structured form of qualitative research which comes closest to being a 'method'
Pragmatic approach	Here, elements of all the above approaches are selected eclectically and in respect of their value to the research objective. Is commonly used in healthcare research

These approaches do not tend to contain a 'method' of doing qualitative research; rather, they should be seen as 'perspectives'.

■ CHARACTERISTICS OF ETHNOGRAPHY

- Focuses on 'meaning' in the context of behaviour
- Takes the actor's (participant's) point of view
- Studies the actor in their own cultural situation
- Focuses on process instead of structures

- Avoids seeing behaviour in term of stereotypes of behaviour, class, race, etc.
- Generalises from descriptions to theory (is inductive) (Gobo, 2011).

■ CHARACTERISTICS OF PHENOMENOLOGY

Phenomenology seeks to interpret the 'lived' experience of individuals. It is principally different from ethnography in that it is interested in individuals and not in social groups or culture

There are two main approaches within phenomenology, although a pragmatic (mixed) approach can be taken:

Husserlian and Heideggerian approaches

	HUSSERLIAN	HEIDEGGERIAN
Objective/ subjective	Phenomenological reduction (bracketing): researcher tries to be neutral	The researcher exposes their values, experiences, etc. and accepts the impact of these on the research
Analysis	Tries to be objective or at least fully 'auditable'	Tries to be interpretive
Context	Context not important	Context all important
Truth	Aims to expose truth via description	Concerned with interpretation of the human understanding of truth. There are multiple truths or truth has a 'multiplicity of layers' (Campbell and Roden, 2010)
Method	Sees merit in a structured approach with clearly defined methods	No defined method

CHARACTERISTICS OF GROUNDED THEORY

- Seeks to develop theory about social processes.
- The literature is reviewed only after the analysis has been commenced. This is so that the researcher is not influenced by existing knowledge.
- Sampling is determined as the data collection progresses (known as 'theoretical sampling') and ends when there is 'data saturation' (when new data does not add to the developing theory).
- Has stages that are more closely defined than is the case with other qualitative approaches. The analysis of data involves:
  - Open coding – to identify 'categories' (broad terms which summarise parts of the data)
  - Axial coding – to identify links between the categories
  - Selective coding – to find the core (or main) category into which the other categories link.
- Data collection and theory building are concurrent, enabling a 'constant comparative analysis' where the researcher moves between the data and the analysis, constantly developing the analysis and re-checking the data to ensure the analysis reflects the data.

CHARACTERISTICS OF QUALITATIVE APPROACHES

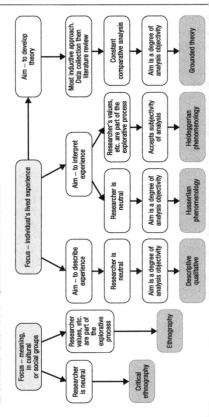

■ AN EXAMPLE OF A PRAGMATIC APPROACH

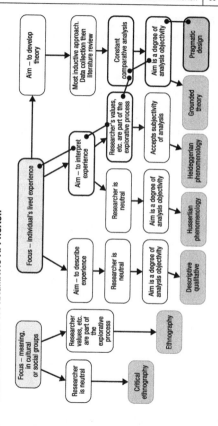

Further reading

Anthony, S. and Jack, S. (2009). 'Qualitative case study methodology in nursing research: an integrative review', *Journal of Advanced Nursing*, 65(6): 1171–1181.

Gobo, G. (2011). 'Ethnography' in *Qualitative Research*, D. Silverman (ed.), Los Angeles: Sage Publications.

Larsson, I. *et al.* (2010). 'Physiotherapists' experience of client participation in physiotherapy interventions: A phenomenographic study', *Advances in Physiotherapy*, 12(4): 217–223.

Livingstone, W. *et al.* (2011). 'A path of perpetual resilience: Exploring the experience of a diabetes-related amputation through grounded theory', *Contemporary Nurse: A Journal for the Australian Nursing Profession*, 39(1): 20–30.

McConnell-Henry, T. *et al.* (2009). 'Husserl and Heidegger: exploring the disparity', *International Journal of Nursing Practice*, 15(1): 7–15.

Smith, J. *et al.* (2011). 'Theoretical versus pragmatic design in qualitative research', *Nurse Researcher*, 18(2): 39–51.

Doing qualitative research

■ STAGES IN THE QUALITATIVE RESEARCH PROCESS

Qualitative research does not have a 'methodology'. However, the following list should at least present a useful guide:

1. Identify the research question.
2. Do a literature review. Note: the purist grounded theory researcher will want to leave the literature review until the data analysis starts.
3. Decide how best to address your research question (e.g. interviews, focus groups, diaries, observation).
4. Decide how you can best recruit participants to the study.
5. Decide on a broad approach to analysis.
6. Consider the ethical implications of what you wish to do.
7. Discuss your research plans with others, make appropriate modifications and obtain ethical approval.
8. Begin collecting the data.
9. Transcribe the data as it comes in.
10. Look at your data as it 'comes in', rather than when you have collected it all.
11. Conduct an 'initial reading' of the text, followed by a closer scrutiny.
12. Identify anything in the text that is interesting, seems 'key', typical, different, odd, etc.
13. Label (code, categorise) the above. These labels will evolve and change as you re-examine the text and look at more text as it comes in.
14. Look for 'negative cases', data that seems to disagree with the developed codes, categories or themes. Ensure these are fully explored.

15. Keep a journal (log, diary). Record every single thought, decision and change of label. What you thought, what you did, why you did it.
16. Regularly review your labels (categories, themes), re-examine text you have already labelled and review the labelling.
17. Identify labels that can be grouped together to form higher level labels.
18. Identify what association or patterns may exist between labels and groups of labels.
19. Identify broad categories of labels that effectively and accurately reflect the data (proto-theories). It is these which will exist as the summary of the analysis and which will be communicated to others when the research is published.
20. Lastly, this is a cognitive exercise, so always 'think'. Never let the 'process' or the 'task' take control. Always think and ask what is this, what is going on here, are my labels (codes, categories) really reflecting the text, are there any patterns here? Always question, 'Am I getting this right?'

Further reading

Banner, D. J. and Albarran, J. W. (2009). 'Computer-assisted qualitative data analysis software: a review', *Canadian Journal of Cardiovascular Nursing*, 19(3): 24–27.

Smith, J. and Firth, J. (2011). 'Qualitative data analysis: the framework approach', *Nurse Researcher*, 18(2): 52–62.

Measuring the trustworthiness of qualitative research

■ TERMS USED

QUALITATIVE TERM	MEANING
Credibility	Similar to 'internal validity'. The degree to which the researcher's interpretation of the data can be justified in the data itself
Transferability	Similar to 'external validity', the degree to which the concepts, constructs or theory generated by the analysis can be applied elsewhere
Dependability	Similar to 'reliability'. If the study was repeated, similar results would be obtained
Plausibility	The degree to which the researcher's interpretation of the data is likely to be realistic given our existing knowledge
Confirmability	The degree to which it is possible to assess whether the findings flow from the data (is the study 'auditable'?)

■ METHODS TO ENSURE TRUSTWORTHINESS

Triangulation	More than one data collection or analysis method
External audits	An audit trail and audit by external body
Member checking	Taking the analysis back to the participants
Negative case analysis	Dealing with cases that do not comply with the main interpretation of the data
Peer debriefing and review	Obtaining feedback
Prolonged engagement/ persistent observation	Spending significant time with participants
Reflexivity (openness about researcher bias)	Evidence of reflection throughout the study

TRUSTWORTHINESS (QUALITY) INDICATORS FOR QUALITATIVE RESEARCH

INDICATOR	COMMENTS
Does the study have a clear focus and goal? Is the research problem clearly stated?	It is important, even with qualitative research that the research has a clear focus
Is there evidence that the research has considered the existing literature? Does the study 'build on' existing knowledge?	Despite being inductive it is still always necessary for the study to build on to existing knowledge and the existing literature should therefore be used at some point in the study
Is the method of recruitment clearly identified?	The study should make it clear how participants were selected, and what the inclusion and exclusion criteria were
Are ethical issues clearly identified?	Were support mechanisms in place for participants?
Is the data collection procedure described clearly?	Both the process and the rationale should be clear and should be compliant with the research question
Is there evidence that data saturation was reached?	This is the point at which new data is not adding anything to the analysis
Method – general: Is there reference to a method or philosophical underpinning?	The research may refer to ethnography, phenomenology, grounded theory, etc. or to an eclectic mix of approaches

INDICATOR	COMMENTS
Method – focus: Does the research make it clear whether the focus is on individual lived experience or to group, culture or societal function?	There is a fundamental difference between trying to interpret lived experience (as in phenomenology) and trying to examine or interpret th meaning in social groups (defining the social group by the meaning individuals have in it), as in ethnography
Method – bracketing: Is it clear whether the researcher tried to be neutral (bracketing) or to be open about values and other attributes?	We need to be clear about whether the researcher tried to be neutral (as in unbiased) or whether they openly accepted their values, experience, assumptions, etc. and used these (purposely) to influence the research
Has the researcher used one or more methods to ensure trustworthiness?	For example, triangulation, audit
Is there an audit trail?	The researcher should have kept a log of each stage in the research process and each stage in the interpretation (cognitive) of the data
Analysis method	It should be possible to obtain a cle picture about how the data was analysed. For example, were codes themes or categories developed from the data?

Further reading

Curtin, M. and Fossey, E. (2007). 'Appraising the trustworthiness of qualitative studies: guidelines for occupational therapists', *Australian Occupational Therapy Journal*, 54(2): 88–94.

Research ethics

■ PRINCIPLES COMMON TO ALL GUIDANCE ON RESEARCH ETHICS

- Planned research must be subject to review by the appropriate research ethics committee.
- Research should be of good quality and be capable of meeting its aims.
- Potential harm must be identified.
- There must be informed and voluntary consent.
- Confidentiality and anonymity must be respected.
- Data should be held securely (data protection).
- Participants have the right to withdraw from the study at any time, without giving a reason and without prejudicing their care or treatment.

■ RESEARCH ON CHILDREN AND VULNERABLE PEOPLE

This area is legally and ethically complex. It is important to obtain authoritative advice and appropriate approval before involving children and vulnerable people in research.

- Parents can sometimes consent for children who may not be able to consent for themselves.
- In cases which exceed minimal risk, parental consent may not be legally valid.

- Children may themselves be able to consent in law (Children Act 1989).
- The child's withdrawal of consent may indicate their lawful ability to consent and so signify the loss of that consent.
- It is good practice to seek consent from children of any age.
- Vulnerable people may not be able to provided informed, voluntary consent.
- Children and vulnerable people may need time to conside consenting to research involvement and will need information provided to them in a form that they will be able to understand.

List of available guidance

British Psychological Society – ethics and standards
http://www.bps.org.uk/what-we-do/ethics-standards/
ethics-standards

General Medical Council – research guidance
http://www.gmc-uk.org/guidance/ethical_guidance/5991.asp

Medical Research Council – ethics and research guidance
http://www.mrc.ac.uk/Ourresearch/Ethicsresearchguidance/
index.htm

NHS National Research Ethics Service
http://www.nres.nhs.uk/applications/is-your-project-research

RCN Research ethics guide
http://www.rcn.org.uk/development/
researchanddevelopment/rs/publications_and_position_
statements/research_ethics_guidance

Relevant law

Children Act 1989
http://www.legislation.gov.uk/ukpga/1989/41/contents

Human Rights Act 1998
http://www.legislation.gov.uk/ukpga/1998/42/contents

Human Tissue Act 2004
http://www.legislation.gov.uk/ukpga/2004/30/contents

Further reading

Williams, J. R. (2008). 'The Declaration of Helsinki and public health . . . original declaration reproduced in full with permission of the World Medical Association', *Bulletin of the World Health Organization*, 86(8): 650–652.

World Medical Association (1964). *Declaration of Helsinki*, Helsinki: World Medical Association.

Implementing published research

Implementing research in healthcare is always a collaborative venture.

■ INITIAL WORK

Be sure of your 'case' by responding to the following questions:

  What does this research suggest in terms of practice change?
  What exactly is the evidence put forward by the research?
  What are the limitations of this research?
  What contradictory research exists on the subject?

- What would be the impact of implementing the research
- What are the risks of:
  - Implementing this change in practice
  - Removing the existing practice?

■ MOVING FORWARD

- Discuss the research with colleagues, informally.
- Get feedback by presenting your ideas regarding the research at a research seminar or similar event.
- Have informal discussions with the chair of the practice implementation (or similar) group.
- Identify the staff who would be affected by the change in practice and keep them informed – allow them to voice their views and to be involved.
- Have the practice implementation group (or similar) formally consider your proposals.
- Open meetings for clinical or other staff to discuss the project.
- Respond to feedback and work to develop an implementation strategy.
- Ensure everyone who needs to know, or thinks they need to know, does know.
- Ensure you have formal permission to go ahead.
- Evaluate the changes and document these.

■ LASTLY

- Be patient, listen to concerns, be prepared to re-think the project if necessary.
- Publish the results of the implementation so that others can benefit from what you have achieved.

Further reading

Stewart, E. (2006). 'Nursing guidelines: Development of catheter care guidelines for Guy's and St Thomas'', *British Journal of Nursing*, 15(8): 420.

Getting involved in research

Research is almost always a collaborative activity. Good research is generally expensive and requires a collaborative effort to obtain funding.

■ BACKGROUND WORK

- Make contact with people already involved in research:
  - There might be an interest group in the NHS Trust.
  - There will certainly be a research implementation group, a practice implementation or procedure group.
- Keep in touch with your university.
- Discuss your research interests with the staff known to you at your university.
- Consider doing a research degree – MRes, MPhil or PhD.
- Join a journal club, research seminar group, etc.
- Be actively involved in subject area groups (cystic fibrosis society, etc.).
- Get to know how your local research ethics committee works.

■ MOVING FORWARD

- Join an existing research group as a junior member.
- Establish a track record and a publishing record as a junior member of one or more research teams.

- Get involved in research grant applications.
- Look for opportunities to share in a grant submission.
- Look to becoming a more senior member of a research team and towards initiating (being the lead member) of a small grant submission.

Be positive and collaborative, don't expect it to be easy, and never give up.

■ RESEARCH DEGREES

Consider reading for a research degree when:

- You need one for your career.
- You know as much as anyone else but you want to take your area of interest further.

MRes (master of research)	Provides research training. Can be used as a 'soft' entry to PhD – where the research training element of the PhD would not need to be repeated	FT – 1 year PT – 2 years
MPhil (master of philosophy)	Essentially, a small PhD. Useful where you know that you will not need a full PhD	FT – 2 years PT – 3 years
PhD (doctor of philosophy)	A UK PhD comprises research training modules plus independent research and creation of a thesis	FT – 3 years PT – 5 years

Publishing research

■ SECTIONS IN A RESEARCH THESIS OR REPORT

The following sections usually provide the structure:
1. Abstract
2. Introduction
3. Literature review
4. Methods (including ethics)
5. Results
6. Discussion of results
7. Conclusion
8. References
9. Appendices

■ PUBLISHING RESEARCH

- Identify two or three journals with which you are 'comfortable' and which are suitable for your research area.
- Read research reports and become familiar with the way they are written in your chosen journals.
- Get help, peer support and peer review, and join a 'journal club'.
- Your article/report should:
  - Have a clear focus
  - Contain a single 'trajectory' (be 'about' something)
  - Communicate a message clearly
  - Have a clear purpose
  - 'Flow' logically.

Use the literature to support your arguments – not to create arguments or discussion.

- Be balanced and fair; make sure your own arguments are supported in some way.
- Be positive if you can.
- Make your discussion interesting.
- Don't rush it, submit it only when it is 'word-perfect'.
- Pay attention to grammar, etc.
- Make sure there are no errors (referencing, etc.).
- Ask: 'Would I want to read this?'

Lastly:

- Don't give up – feedback from the journal may seem very negative, but respond to it and resubmit your work – again and again if necessary.

Further reading

Oermann, M. H. *et al.* (2006). 'Presenting research to clinicians: strategies for writing about research findings'. *Nurse Researcher*, 13(4): 66–74.

Glossary

Actor Syn. 'research participant'.

Assumptions (data assumptions) The criteria that data must meet in order for a test to be run on that data.

Audit trail Clear documentation of each step in the research process.

Axial coding Identifying relationships between the identified categories (or themes) assigned to qualitative data.

Axiology The study of values.

Between group (difference, variance, effects) The 'effect' (difference) found between (usually) the control group and the intervention group.

Bias The unwitting misrepresentation of data which causes the results to lack validity (be untrue). Bias is generally dealt with by blinding and by randomisation.

Bivariate A design containing two variables (often seen in correlation studies).

Blinding Where the researcher and/or the participant are unaware of whether they are in the intervention or the control group.

Categorical variable A variable in the form of categories (yes, no). Syn. 'nominal data'.

Conditions Groups within an independent variable (SEX – male, female).

Confidence interval A statistical test of how likely it is that a measure (e.g. the mean) taken from a sample would be found in the population.

Confirmability The degree to which it is possible to assess whether the findings flow from the data.

Constant comparative method Where the researcher analyses the text on a continuous basis, as new data is brought in and by constantly examining and re-examining the text in relation to the developing themes or categories.

Constructivist (interpretive) paradigm The notion that much of the world is 'open to interpretation', that there is no objective truth or measurable facts and that instead, 'truth' is something that we perceive to be there.

Content analysis An overarching term meaning any qualitative analysis. Sometimes meaning a more structured analysis of qualitative data.

Continuous scale Data existing as a scale and where the difference between two points on the scale is not meaningful.

control, control group	The group to which the intervention being tested is *not* applied.
correlation (correlational study)	The degree of interrelationship between two variables.
credibility	Similar to 'internal validity'. The degree to which the researcher's interpretation of the data can be justified in the data itself.
data saturation	The point at which new data from participants fails to add anything useful to the analysis. Signals the completion of the data collection.
dependability	Similar to 'reliability'. If the study was repeated, similar results would be obtained.
dependent variable	The variable that is being tested or acted upon by the independent variable.
descriptive statistics	Descriptive statistics describe the data, rather than drawing inferences from the data. Mean, mode and median are examples of descriptive statistics.
descriptive study	Seeks to describe what already exists. Syn. 'retrospective study'.
design	The plan for the study.
discourse analysis	The way language is used to represent social or cultural understanding of a phenomenon.

Discrete (data) — Syn. 'nominal' or 'categorical'.

Distribution (normal distribution) — The distribution of scores. A normal distribution produces a bell-shaped curve when charted.

Epistemology — The theory of knowledge.

Ethnography — The meaning people have in being a part of a culture and a member of society.

Experiment — Research which seeks to cause an effect which can then be measured

Factor — A group or condition within an independent variable. Such groups categorical.

Framework analysis — A process of managing the coding qualitative data and which involves mapping of themes to cases.

Grounded theory — First devised by Glaser and Strauss (1967). Is characterised by the use constant comparative analysis and generation of theory inductively.

Groups — 'Group' is a loose term which usual refers to a design condition.

Hegemony — Imperial dominance. Used by qualitative researchers to describe dominance of quantitative research (the hegemony of positivism).

Heideggerian hermeneutic phenomenology	From Martin Heidegger (1889–1976). Sees truth as having no objective reality. The researcher's values are allowed to impact on the study.
Hermeneutic cycle (hermeneutics)	The subjective interpretation of the participant's experience (though open to audit).
Husserlian phenomenology	After Edmund Husserl, 1859–1938. The researcher tries to maintain a neutral position ('bracketing') during the data collection and analysis.
Hypothesis	A statement of the expected outcome of the research.
Independent variable	The 'treatment' variable. The variable introduced in an experiment to produce a change in the dependent variable.
Inductive	From data to theory.
Inferential statistics	Inferential statistics are so named because they draw inferences from the data. Inferential statistics are generally used to identify probability.
Interactionism	A term introduced by Herbert Blumer (1900–1987). A form of fieldwork which can be seen to form the basis of ethnography.

Interpretive paradigm	An acceptance that truth is subjective
Interval data	A continuous scale (as in a 1–100 scale) where the difference between two points on the scale is not meaningful.
Intervention	The effect of the independent variable on the dependent variable.
Likert scale	A scale of 1–5 containing textual labels.
Member checking	The sharing of the summary or the analysis of the participant's data with the participant.
Meta-analysis	An analysis run on pooled data from more than one study. Meta-analyses are most commonly seen in systematic reviews.
Mixed methods	The use of two of more methods to achieve trustworthiness.
Multivariate	Many variables (or generally, more than two).
Negative case analysis	A deliberate attempt to deal with aspects of the data which do *not* agree with the developing findings during the data analysis.
Nominal	Categories (such as yes, no).

Non-parametric statistics	A group of statistical procedures which can be run on ordinal (non-continuous) data and where data is not normally distributed).
One-tailed, two tailed	The prediction of an effect in one direction only (one-tailed) or in either direction (two-tailed).
Ontology	Theory of meaning.
Open coding	Categories (themes) in the data are identified.
Ordinal	Originally meaning data placed in order but generally meaning data from a short scale or a non-continuous scale. For example, a 1–5 Likert scale.
Parametric statistics	Parametric statistics are a range of statistical procedures usually used on interval and ratio data. The data have to have the following characteristics (often called 'assumptions'): (a) the dependent variable is at the interval or ratio level of measurement; (b) the dependent variable is approximately normally distributed; (c) there is similar variance between the two groups (homogeneity of variance).
Peer de-briefing and peer review	A process by which people not directly involved in the study are able to examine it.

Phenomenology In practice, phenomenology focuses on the interpretation of the 'lived experience' of individuals.

Plausibility The degree to which the researcher's interpretation of the data is likely to realistic given our existing knowledge

Population The potential data set to which the sample relates.

Positivist paradigm (positivism) The notion that the world is chiefly a objective and measurable place. Syn 'traditional science'.

Post hoc tests Post hoc tests such as Scheffé's and Tukey's are run after analyses involving more than two conditions to identify effects in respect of each condition.

Post-modern (post-structural) A belief that there is no coherent way of explaining phenomena in structural terms.

Post-test The testing carried out after the 'treatment' (intervention).

Pragmatic paradigm Where dealing with the research question is considered to be more important than adhering to a pure methodological approach.

Pre-test The testing carried out before the 'treatment' (intervention).

Pre-test/post-test design	A study which in which testing takes place prior to the intervention and after the intervention – in order to determine the effect of the intervention.
Probability (p. value)	The identified risk that the observed effect was caused by chance alone.
Prolonged engagement	An aspect of the quality of research (trustworthiness). The longer the time the researcher spends with participants the richer and more understood will be the data and the interpretation of it.
Q-Q plot	The Q-Q plot is a graphical illustration of the degree to which data is normally distributed.
Radical (critical) interpretivism	A form of phenomenology which seeks not merely to describe experiences but to change them. Most clearly seen in research on feminism and social justice.
Random, randomisation	A process of recruiting participants or allocating participants to groups, where potential participants have an equal chance of being selected.
Randomised control trial (RCT)	An experiment which includes randomisation, a control group and (usually) blinding.

Ranked data (ranking)	Data that is put in order (as in 12, 23 45, 67, 99) or that already exists as ordered data.
Ratio data	Data existing on a continuous scale with no end points (e.g. blood pressure).
Realism	Belief in a stable and objective reality
Recruitment	The process of including participants in a qualitative study. In quantitative studies, the word 'sampling' is used.
Reflexivity	Researcher self-scrutiny.
Related (design)	Where the same individuals (or matched, paired individuals) are tested on more than one occasion.
Relativism	Belief in a socially constructed reality
Reliability	The degree to which the same result would be obtained if the study were be repeated.
Rigour	The quality of research.
Robust	A general term for the quality of a research study.
Sample	The part of the population of cases used within the research study.
Sampling	The procedure (method) used to produce the sample.
Scale	Any data that is distributed between two points.

elective coding
The process of identifying the 'core' or central category (theme) from those identified during the analysis of qualitative data.

ignificance (level)
Syn. 'probability'.

tandard deviation
A measure of dispersion around the mean, or the within-group variability.

urvey
A descriptive study having just one 'group'.

urvival analysis
These are a range of statistical procedures, including the Kaplan-Meier survival procedure designed to identify the impact of an independent variable on 'survival'. The survival variable is time.

ystematic review
A meta-analysis of pooled research data from several studies.

ext
Used by qualitative researchers, meaning 'data'.

hematic analysis
The development of themes in qualitative analysis.

heoretical eneralisability
The way in which concepts and theories derived from qualitative research can be generalised.

hick description
The production of a detailed description of the qualitative data, often with quotes from the transcripts.

Transferability	Similar to 'external validity', the degree to which the concepts, constructs or theory generated by the qualitative analysis can be applied elsewhere.
Triangulation (triangulation studies)	A technique where more than one method is used to collect or analyse data. Is used to enhance the credibi or trustworthiness of a qualitative study.
Trustworthiness	The quality or robustness of qualitat research.
Univariate	One variable. A univariate analysis i an analysis run on just one variable.
Unrelated (unrelated design)	Data is collected from two or more separate groups of participants whe differences between the groups are hypothesised.
Validity	Internal validity: the degree to which the researcher's interpretation of the data can be justified in the data itself. The degree to which the data what we think it is (that it is true or 'valid'). External validity: the degree to which the results of the study can be generalised to the relevant population.

Variable	Literally, something that varies. In practice, it is either the thing that we are measuring (dependent variable) or the thing that is causing the effect (independent variable).
Within groups (difference, variance, effects)	The amount of variation (difference) that exists within one variable.

Further reading

Jolley, M. J. (2010). *Introducing research and evidence based practice for nurses.* Harlow: Pearson.

Websites

NHS Health Research Authority: seeks to protect and promote the interests of patients and the public in health research.
http://www.hra.nhs.uk/

NHS National Institute for Health Research: supports NHS research.
http://www.nihr.ac.uk/Pages/default.aspx

References

Campbell, S. and Roden, J. (2010). 'Research approaches for novice nephrology nurse researchers', *Renal Society of Australasia Journal*, 6(3): 114–120.

Glaser, B. G. and Strauss, A. (1967). *The discovery of grounded theory: strategies for qualitative research*, Chicago: Aldine.

Gobo, G. (2011). 'Ethnography' in *Qualitative research*, D. Silverman (ed.), Los Angeles: Sage Publications.

Magilvy, J. K. and Thomas, E. (2009). 'Scientific inquiry. A first qualitative project: qualitative descriptive design for novice researchers', *Journal for Specialists in Pediatric Nursing*, 14(4): 298–300.

Whiting, L. S. (2008). 'Semi-structured interviews: guidance for novice researchers', *Nursing Standard*, 22(23): 35–40.